Osteoporosis

I0417480

Causes, Symptoms and Prevention

RON KNESS

No part of this book may be reproduced, stored in a retrieval system, or transmitted in any form or by any means, electronic, mechanical, photocopying, recording, scanning, or otherwise, without the prior written permission of the publisher, except for the inclusion of brief quotations in a review.

This book is for **personal use only**.

Copyright © 2017 Ron Kness

All rights reserved.

ISBN-13: 978-1544231631

ISBN-10: 1544231636

1

Contents

Disclaimer

This publication is for informational purposes only and is not intended as medical advice. Medical advice should always be obtained from a qualified medical professional for any health conditions or symptoms associated with them.

Every possible effort has been made in preparing and researching this material. We make no warranties with respect to the accuracy, applicability of its contents or any omissions.

See your healthcare professional before starting any diet, health or exercise program!

Introduction

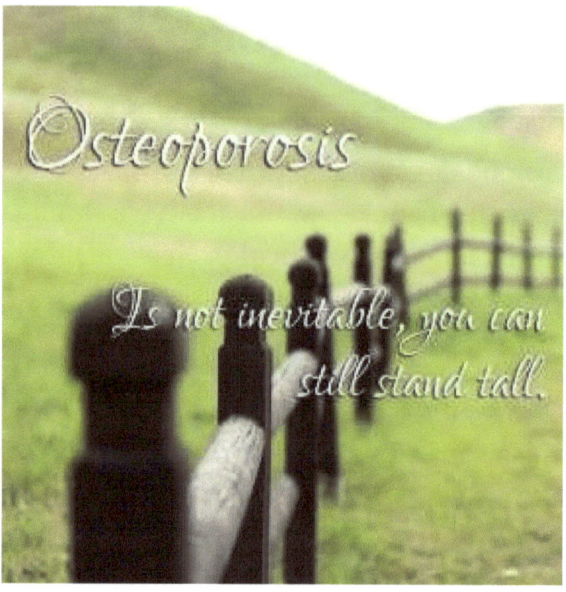

Osteoporosis, also known as 'Brittle Bone Disease' has been referred to as 'The Silent Epidemic'.

Hundreds of thousands of spontaneous fractures and crush fractures occur every year due to the "bone thinning" that results from the condition known as osteoporosis. Although the whole skeleton is affected, areas commonly affected by fractures are the hip, spine and wrist.

As a result of this condition, height loss and stooping can occur. This can subsequently lead to the vertebra in the spine collapsing.

Predisposing Factors Include:

- A deficiency in vitamin D, very common in modern western society.

- Eating fat-free diets.

- Drinking 2 or more cups of coffee every day can greatly diminish bone mineral density in women. For men, alcohol is the major culprit.

- Following are some health tips that can be undertaken by almost anyone to help maintain a healthy bone structure.

Natural Remedies

- Comfrey root is well known for promoting growth of bone cells.

- Calendula or Marigold encourages granulation.

- Calcium metabolism is assisted by Horsetail.

- Cayenne Pepper offers a positive effect on the circulation in order to transport nutrients throughout the body.

- Fenugreek tea is helpful.

- Bee propolis has a reputation for helping bone tissue regenerate.

Dietary Recommendations

- Eat plenty of green veggies and fresh fruit.

- Fish and fish oils included in the diet.

- Avoid excessive quantities of heavy meat meals as they interfere with calcium metabolism.

- Avoid excess salt as it can aggravate bone loss and causes phosphorus and calcium to be excreted through the kidneys.

- Slippery Elm and Irish Moss can be taken for their mineral content.

- Fresh, unadulterated water should be consumed regularly.

- Beneficial supplements include: Vitamin E, Magnesium, Vitamin B12, Zinc, Vitamin D and Vitamin C.

Herbal Teas

Mix together equal parts of Nettles, Alfalfa and Comfrey leaves. Dose is 2 teaspoons to each cup of boiling water; allow to steep for 5 to 15 minutes and drink 1 cup, 3 times a day.

Make a tea with 3 parts oats, 1 part Horsetail, 1 part Marigold petals and 2 parts Comfrey leaves to each cup of boiling water. Infuse for 5 to 15 minutes and drink one cup freely.

Mature Women Most at Risk

Osteoporosis is particularly prevalent after menopause. Women over 50 are the demographic which most suffer from measured bone loss. Reduced estrogen levels are believed to speed up the rate of reduction in bone mass.

Our bones act as a store of calcium. When calcium is needed for critical body tasks not being supplied by dietary intake, the body will temporarily 'rob' some calcium from the bones. This will be replenished when conditions allow.

Pregnant and lactating women have a great requirement for calcium placed on their bodies to nourish their growing child, before and after the birth. As such, their bone density can be very compromised, especially if their diet is lacking in any of the nutrients necessary for bone growth.

It is very likely that some of the loss of bone density which becomes obvious after menopause is instigated due to the rigors of child-bearing and rearing.

Supportive Measures

Our skeletal system needs to be functioning in an optimal manner every day in order for us to perform at our healthy best. If our bones become brittle or weak due to a lack of mineral absorption from a poor diet, we will suffer the effects in many ways.

One of the best things you can do is exercise in the sun! Spending more time in the sun helps to obtain natural vitamin D absorption. If you are a smoker, STOP! As well as improving your overall health it will allow for optimum mineral absorption to rejuvenate your skeletal system.

What Causes Osteoporosis?

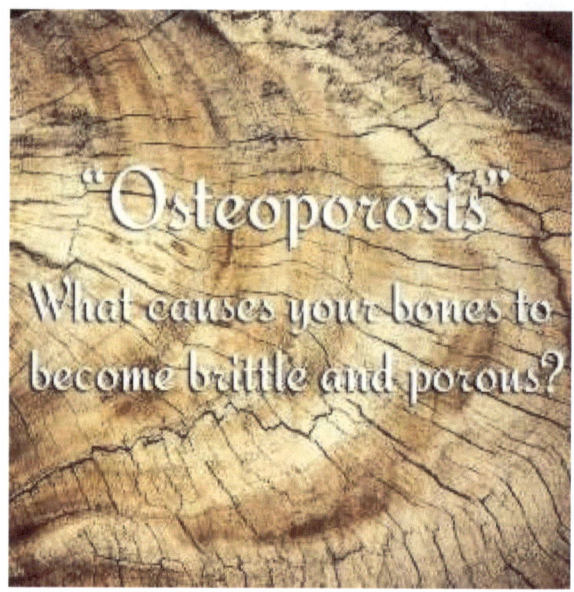

Osteoporosis is the name of a condition which causes weakening of the bones, but as this 'condition' is becoming more common today, people are beginning to ask, 'what causes osteoporosis in the first place?'

Bones are not solid, they are porous and any reduction in bone density means less bone and more 'pores'. Testing for osteoporosis is a measure of the density of our bones. When a person's bone density drops below a specified level, the subject is diagnosed as having osteoporosis.

There are many reasons why people suffer from osteoporosis. One of these is the imbalance that occurs between new bone production made by osteoblasts and bone reabsorption from osteoclasts. When the rate of bone reabsorption is higher than the rate of bone tissue creation, demineralization and bone thinning will start to occur.

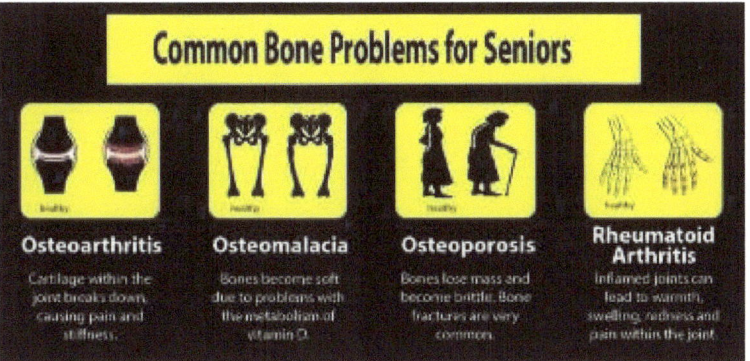

Here are the causes and predisposing factors of bone thinning or osteoporosis:

1. Gender

Studies show that women are at a much greater risk of developing osteoporosis than men. Large hormonal changes which women undergo have great effects on their bone density. A rapid decrease in their estrogen levels, such as occurs during menopause, directly results in a decrease in bone density.

Furthermore, the effects of pregnancy and lactation make large demands on the minerals and vitamins essential to bone health and strength, particularly calcium and magnesium.

In men, testosterone aids in keeping bones healthy and the risk of osteoporosis increases if testosterone level decreases.

2. Vitamin D

Vitamin D is one of the essential vitamins needed for calcium absorption in the intestines to promote the normal growth of bones. Low levels of vitamin D impair the body's normal absorption of calcium and accelerate osteoporosis.

3. Parathyroid Hormone

Parathyroid Hormone is an important regulator of calcium in the blood. When there is a deficiency of calcium, the body secretes the parathyroid hormone to increase the levels of calcium in the blood.

The calcium is taken from the stored calcium in the bones. If the parathyroid glands are overactive and the hormone is released in excessive levels a continual leaching effect will occur, which in turn makes the bones brittle and prone to osteoporosis.

4. Bone Formation and Bone Resorption Imbalance

The most common cause of osteoporosis, especially as a person ages, is the imbalance between bone formation and bone resorption. Usually, the body compensates for bone loss by forming new bone matter, in a natural cycle.

However, as the person ages this balance between bone formation and bone resorption tends to skew. Aging affects the body by failing to readily form new bone or increasingly absorbing too much old bone.

5. Diet

Diet is a contributing factor in the development and cause of osteoporosis. To prevent osteoporosis, it is important to acquire and absorb the necessary vitamins and minerals that promote healthy bone growth.

The macro component that most people are aware of is the need for calcium.

Calcium is a vital mineral needed for the proper functioning of organs. Calcium is stored in the bones. However, whenever blood levels of calcium are depleted, the body reabsorbs calcium from the bones, hopefully only temporarily.

Many people are less aware that magnesium is essential for calcium absorption by the body. If magnesium is not present calcium cannot be absorbed and will simply be excreted.

Nutrition must also include vitamin D since it also helps the body to absorb calcium efficiently. Without enough vitamin D, the body cannot absorb calcium from the diet no matter how much calcium is available.

Other vitamins which promote bone growth are vitamin K and vitamin B.

In addition, it is important to limit the intake of substances that hinder bone growth such as caffeine and excessive protein. These can cause the body to excrete calcium and reduce the body's capacity to absorb available calcium.

6. Sedentary lifestyle

A sedentary lifestyle can cause or hasten osteoporosis. For bones to repair and replace themselves requires weight-bearing, or else there is no impetus for the body to increase bone density. Standing for at least half an hour a day is important for strong, healthy bones.

Two hours is even better. Simply standing can be quite boring; a daily walk can provide the needed weight-bearing requirement plus provide added cardio benefits.

No Single Cure

There are many factors that cause a reduction in bone density and contribute to the development of osteoporosis such as age, gender, physiological factors, predisposing conditions, lifestyle and diet. Some of these are obviously pre-determined and beyond your control.

However, variables such as diet and exercise and medication are very much up to you and should be the focus of your efforts in controlling osteoporosis.

What Are the Symptoms of Osteoporosis?

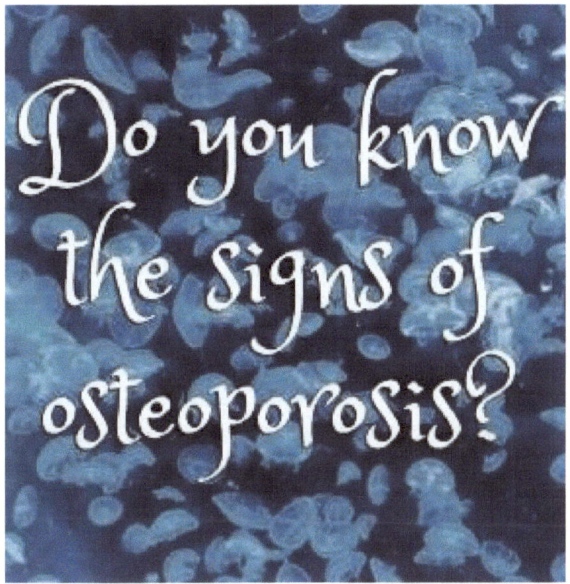

There are many factors which can contribute to osteoporosis, and the condition may be well advanced before obvious signs and symptoms are visible. A person leading a relatively sedentary or non-physical lifestyle may not be aware of their bone loss and may put down any noticeable physical differences down to just getting older.

There are a few signs and symptoms to be on the lookout for, including the following.

Symptoms of Osteoporosis

Bone Breakage or Fractures

The most obvious symptom (and how many find out they have developed osteoporosis) is too often from the result of a bone breakage.

This can be in areas and joints that carry a major share of the load such as the hip, spine or wrist. These fractures may occur though seemingly minor actions such as stepping off a curb or lifting something too heavy.

The person may experience pain and wonder why! When x-rays are taken to diagnose the pain, a bone fracture is often found and the level of bone density loss is apparent to the doctor.

Curvature of The Spine

Another obvious sign of osteoporosis is a marked curvature of the spine. Loss of skeletal strength results in a less than ideal posture.

Additionally, an injury to multiple vertebra of the spine can compress the vertebra together also resulting in a pronounced curvature of the spine.

The curving of the upper back was once known as a dowager's hump. Dowager means an elderly woman or widow. This is because, although anyone can be affected by osteoporosis, most sufferers were and are women, particularly older women.

Loss of Height

A loss of height occurs together with a stooped posture. This may be due to compression fractures in the spine, as well as the reduction of the vertebra mass and the shrinking of the gel-filled disks between them.

Joint Pain

Sometimes osteoporosis contributes to joint pain and swelling that is easily confused with arthritis. Due to personal misdiagnosis, many osteoporosis cases get worse before medical help is sought. Pain and swelling of the joints should be brought to a doctor's attention to determine the cause and appropriate remedial action and treatment.

Dental Problems

Research has shown that many people suffering with teeth loss and periodontal disease are also diagnosed with osteoporosis. The studies showed that people who had osteoporosis were at a much higher risk of having periodontal disease.

There is a higher incidence of both periodontal disease and osteoporosis in post-menopausal women, compared to other demographics.

Other Contributing Risk Factors

Apart from the age aspect, some people may be more prone to developing osteoporosis due to other risk factors.

Some risk factors that could contribute to developing osteoporosis are:

- Constitution – the build of the body is a factor in developing osteoporosis; those that are thinner or more slightly built are more prone to this condition.

- Gender – osteoporosis affects many more women than men, and to a larger degree.

- Physical Activity – people who are physically active are less likely to develop osteoporosis than those who are inactive.

- Genetics – studies show that children who have parents with osteoporosis are more likely to develop osteoporosis as they age.

Osteoporosis can occur and develop even while noticeable symptoms are absent.

Often, we tend to take for granted such symptoms or mistake them for something else. This gives more time for the condition to go undiagnosed and for the bones to deteriorate further.

Prevention is better than cure, so start eating a bone healthy diet and exercise regularly out in the sun!

Can You Reverse Osteoporosis?

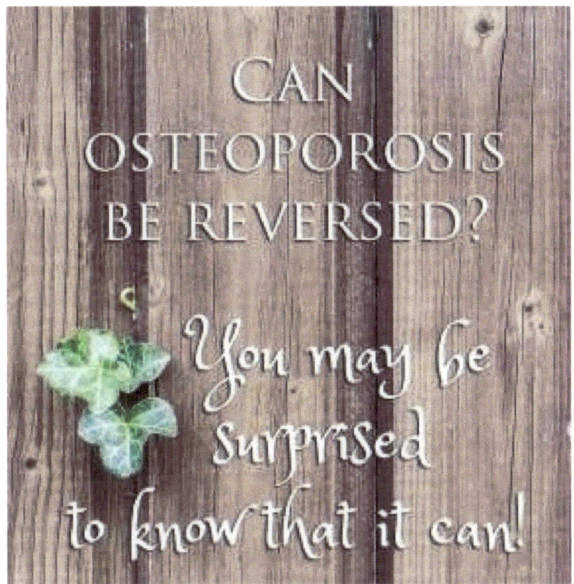

Osteoporosis is a condition in which the density of the body's bones decreases below what is considered a normal or safe limit. Proactive, preventative action can help delay the onset and reduce the degree of any osteoporosis that may later occur.

While prevention is the ideal, the reality is that many people have a diagnosis of osteoporosis thrust upon them with no warning or expectation. Upon being diagnosed with osteoporosis an obvious first question is – can it be reversed?

Once osteoporosis is confirmed, action can also be taken to prevent it from worsening or at the very least limiting the rate of bone mass reduction. With proper management, bone density can be increased, which means effectively reversing osteoporosis.

Here are some useful tips to prevent or "reverse" osteoporosis:

Avoid or reduce intake of cola drinks.

A study done by the renowned Tufts University displayed a distinct correlation between cola drink consumption and hip bone density in women. The more cola this group of participants consumed, the greater the bone density loss in that area.

Caffeine is not bone-friendly.

Caffeine makes you lose calcium through your urine. For every cup of coffee you drink, you can lose 150 mg of calcium. Try tea instead!

Cut out the antacids.

Acid blocking drugs or antacids are predominantly used to treat heartburn and gastritis. Stomach acid is a necessary ingredient to enable calcium, magnesium, and zinc to be absorbed. These minerals are all essential to maintaining and increasing bone density.

Taking excessive antacids decreases the volume of stomach acids and will result in poor absorption of these minerals, thereby increasing the risk of osteoporosis.

Too much protein is not ideal.

Excess protein intake causes the body and blood to be slightly acidic which causes calcium to be excreted via the urine in an attempt to balance the pH levels. 2-4 ounces of lean protein per meal is the recommended allowance.

Get calcium – the right kind of calcium.

Not all calcium supplements are the same. Calcium carbonate is poorly absorbed by the body, although some sellers may claim otherwise. In addition, calcium carbonate causes a reduction in stomach acids which adversely affects calcium uptake. The best kinds of calcium are calcium citrate and calcium hydroxyapatite.

Vitamin D

Vitamin D is a very important vitamin for skeletal strength. Vitamin D helps the bones absorb calcium and the best way to obtain this essential vitamin is through exposing yourself to the sun's rays. The safest way to acquire vitamin D without risking skin cancer is exposure to the sun early in the morning before the heat of the day.

If your lifestyle or work limits your access to sunlight, vitamin D supplementation is readily available from pharmacies and health stores.

Monitor your hormones.

Hormonal fluctuation and decline is the most common cause of osteoporosis among menopausal women and andropausal men. Hormone imbalance accelerates bone loss so maintaining hormonal levels is important to maintain bone density and integrity.

Thyroid and parathyroid hormone levels can also contribute to bone loss. Hormone levels should be monitored so that supplementation can be given if required to minimize effects on bone density.

People who have healthy diets and engage in physical activity are far less likely to develop osteoporosis than inactive people who eat unhealthy foods. Our lifestyle contributes greatly to maintaining skeletal strength and preventing degeneration in the future.

A healthy diet, frequent and regular exercise and a low stress lifestyle will have a large impact on reversing osteoporosis. The same simple, healthy life choices that help reduce the risk of lifestyle diseases will also help keep osteoporosis at bay!

How to Prevent Osteoporosis

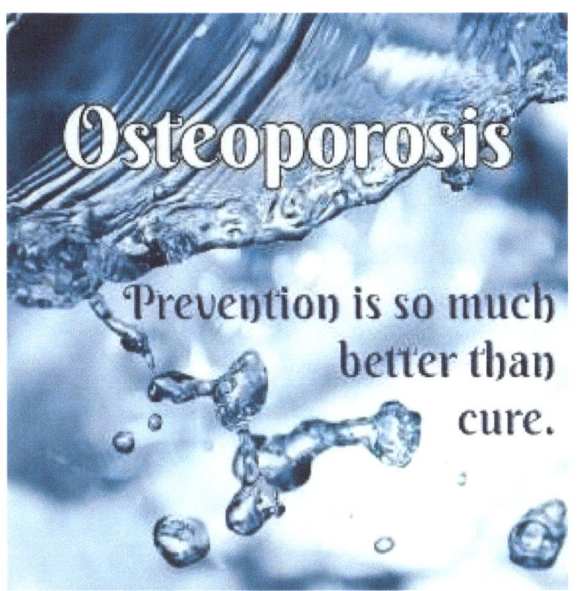

Prevention is far better than later searching for an osteoporosis cure or treatment. Saving your bones now is easier than trying to rebuild lost bone later and it is never too early to begin. Below is a list of tips that will help strengthen bones and help prevent developing osteoporosis.

Calcium and Magnesium

Calcium is the macro mineral that is considered so crucial for the development and overall health of bones. However, you also need magnesium, vitamin D and trace elements for your body to be able to utilize the calcium needed.

Most people take calcium supplements but forget to take other supplements to prevent osteoporosis. Without the other necessary elements, excess calcium cannot be utilized and will be uselessly excreted from the body.

Almost 99% of calcium in the body can be found in the teeth and bones. However, the rest of the body also has need of calcium and will take it from the skeleton if blood calcium is low. Our body uses and loses calcium through our hair, nails, skin, feces and urine. It is very important that we include calcium-rich foods in our diet, such as fresh veggies, greens, beans, dairy, herbs and spices that are calcium-rich.

Weight-bearing Exercises

Spending at least 20 minutes performing weight-bearing exercise daily will greatly help keep the integrity of your bones. Even simply standing for 30 minutes a day is 'weight-bearing'. Your body is supporting your body-weight, which provides the impulsion for your body to increase skeletal mass.

Research has proven that without daily weight-bearing stress being applied to the skeleton, even a large intake of calcium is ineffective and all but useless, as the body will not lay down new bone unless it needs to.

This action is similar to the actions that cause muscle growth – muscle mass increases relative to the loads placed upon them. With the skeleton, however, individual bones do not need to be stressed or loaded. The load placed upon our large leg and hip bones provides the impetus for the body to create bone growth over the whole skeleton.

Your exercise regimen may include running, yoga, tennis and jogging. Domestic chores that involve standing are also weight-bearing exercises.

This includes activities such as ironing (while standing) and gardening, even simply standing and watering your plants.

These kinds of physical activities will give your bones the opportunity to support your body weight, thus encouraging new bone growth.

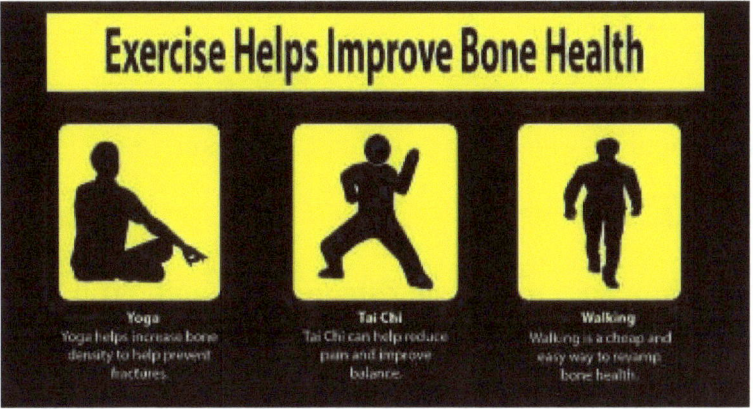

Maintain a Healthy Weight

If you are overweight, you now have another good reason to think about losing any excess pounds. Obese or overweight individuals are at a higher risk of developing osteoporosis.

This may sound strange knowing that 'weight-bearing' is important for healthy bones, however, a survey from NHANES (National Health and Nutrition Examination Survey), showed that obese women were four times more at risk of osteoporosis than women of normal weight. Obese men were five times more likely to have osteoporosis than non-obese men.

Quit Smoking

Smoking affects your health in all areas, including your bone health. Cigarette smoking is known to be a significant contributor towards bone mineral density loss.

A study revealed that 80-year-old smokers were found to have 10% lower bone mineral density than non-smokers. That means that smokers are twice as likely to suffer from spinal fractures, and they also face a 50% higher risk of getting hip fractures.

Another disadvantage of being a smoker is that fractures tend to heal very slowly compared to non-smokers.

Limit Alcohol Intake

If you really want to prevent osteoporosis, and if you tend to over-indulge on alcohol, now is a good time to start reducing your alcohol intake.

Study after study has shown that alcohol consumption can adversely affect bone health. Alcohol has been shown to decrease the production of estrogen. When the estrogen production declines, the process of bone remodeling also slows down which in turn leads to bone loss.

So, if you want to prevent osteoporosis, the best thing you can do is to follow a healthy lifestyle. Eat right, exercise regularly, don't drink or smoke and you'll save your bones naturally!

Vitamins and Minerals for Osteoporosis Prevention

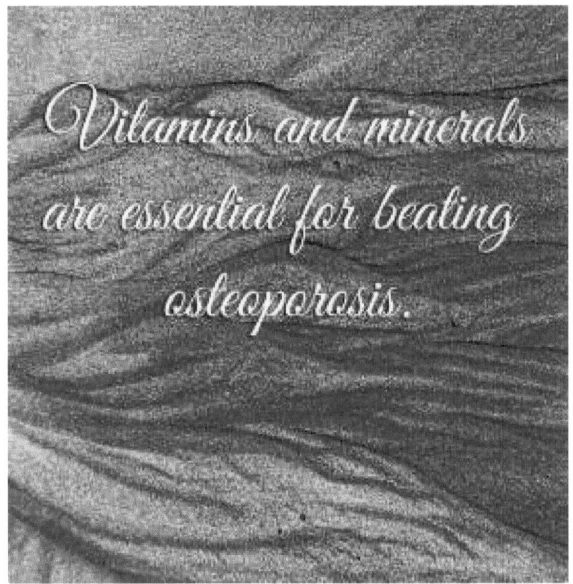

Osteoporosis is a largely preventable disease and there are definitely things you can do to prevent its occurrence. The areas over which we have the most personal impact are diet and exercise. For bone health, the exercise required is weight-bearing exercise.

While aerobic and strength exercise is great for our overall health, what is required to promote bone growth is simply anything that requires us to be standing upright, for at least thirty minutes per day and preferably for two hours.

This assumes that our body has the right materials to create the bone from. Our bones consist mostly of minerals, particularly calcium.

However, to create our bones also requires other minerals and also some vitamins. In the absence of calcium our body cannot create or repair bones. In the absence of the other needed nutrients calcium cannot be utilized for bone creation and excess will be passed from the body.

Those suffering from osteoporosis often show inadequate body levels of zinc, magnesium and vitamin D. Having these essential minerals in balance is a great start to preventing bone loss.

Vitamin D can be obtained by safe exposure of the skin to the sun and also from diet. The other vitamins and minerals needed will need to sourced from the diet. When the essential bone-building nutrients cannot be obtained from dietary sources, supplementation is necessary.

Here are some herbs, teas and foods that contain essential vitamins and minerals that assist in bone building and repair.

Calcium Rich Herbs

The following are herbs that can be easily incorporated into your day either as a tea, tablet, powder, or tincture:

Nettle Tea, Chamomile Tea, Alfalfa, Plantain, Silverweed, Liquorice, Mullein, Meadowsweet, Black Cohosh, Rest Harrow, Dong Quai, Toadflax, Pimpernel, Fenugreek, Fennel, Unicorn Root, Clivers and Shepard's Purse. Irish Moss has a high mineral content.

Calcium Rich Teas

- Incorporating some herbal teas into your diet can be a simple and healthy way to increase your daily calcium levels.

- Liquorice tastes delicious and has a sweet aftertaste so it is nice as a dessert in the evening or afternoon if you are craving something sweet. Be mindful if you have high blood pressure though.

- A cup of Chamomile before bed or when you are feeling anxious will soothe and relax and is great for getting your body prepared to sleep.

- Fennel tea can be made with the seeds from your spice cupboard.

- Nettle tea is high in iron as well and very nutritious.

- Try blending some of these together to make a tasty, customized drink that you will enjoy.

Diet

- Green veggies and fresh raw fruit is ideal. Fish and fish oils are also important.

- Dairy foods contain large amounts of calcium and have long been promoted as a dietary source.

- Osteoporosis is less prevalent in those on a vegetarian diet. It is believed that heavy meat meals inhibit calcium metabolism.

- A high protein diet, however, is beneficial.

Try different non-meat sources such as beans, nuts and organic soy products.

- Avoid alcohol and soft drinks, especially cola drinks.

- Avoid high salt intake as this leads to a loss of phosphorus and calcium through the kidneys, thus placing the skeleton at risk and aggravating bone loss.

Helpful Supplements

When dietary sources may be inadequate, the following are recommended daily:

- Vitamin B6 50mg,

- Zinc 15mg,

- Magnesium citrate 500mg,

- Calcium citrate 1g,

- Vitamin D 1000i.u.,

- Vitamin B12 50mcg,

- Folic Acid 200mcg,

- Vitamin C 500mg-1000mg (although many people are taking much higher amounts of Vitamin C).

- Vitamin A and Boron are also extremely beneficial.

Eating healthy foods that contain the vitamins and minerals you need and exercising is a great start in preventing brittle bones. These are also the areas over which we have the most control.

While we cannot do much about our genetics, we can certainly improve our bone health with good diet and some exercise.

Management of Osteoporosis Pain

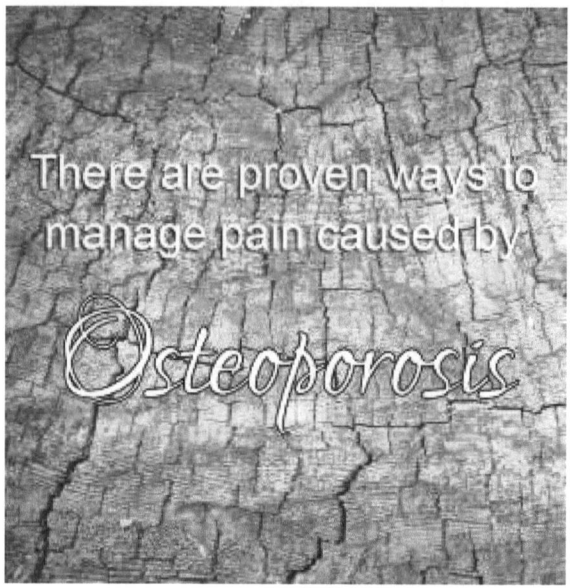

Osteoporosis can cause pain and discomfort for many of those afflicted with the condition. In too many cases sufferers don't realize the pain is due to osteoporosis. This is because until osteoporosis is specifically diagnosed, most people are unaware they have it.

Therefore, they tend to blame their aches on pains on other conditions, such as arthritis, or simply 'back pain'. Often, a diagnosis only occurs following a bone break. Once a diagnosis has been made and acknowledged by the patient, a focus on remedial treatment and pain relief can be undertaken.

As osteoporosis is a very common condition there have been many treatments tried and tested. Listed below are treatment options others have found effective in managing the pain associated with osteoporosis.

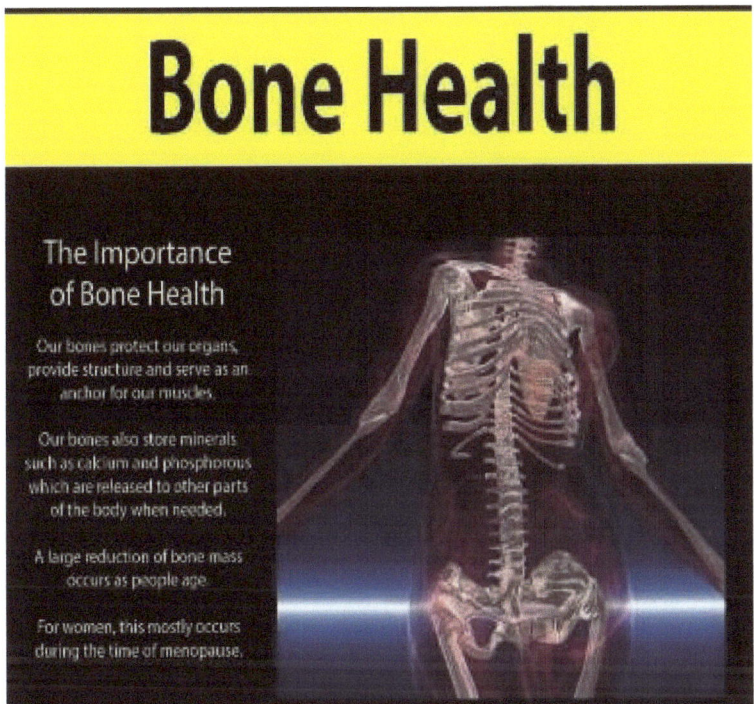

Hot or Cold Treatment

Using either hot or ice packs can be very effective in alleviating pain caused by osteoporosis. If you find yourself feeling stiff in the morning try a warm bath. Warm water can help loosen up the stiffness.

Alternatively, if it is too painful to move, use a cold pack to reduce any joint inflammation and swelling. The use of a cold pack can also help numb the nerves sending the pain signals, which will reduce the intensity of the pain.

You can make your own cold packs by placing frozen beans or peas into a re-sealable plastic bag. This type of home-made ice pack can more easily follow the body shape than many commercial products, allowing the coldness of the pack to penetrate easily into uneven or oddly shaped area.

TENS (Transcutaneous Electrical Nerve Stimulation)

A TENS device makes use of electrical impulses to block pain signals in the body. Electrodes are placed on the skin near the painful area and then a mild electric current is transmitted. This action prevents pain signals from being sent to the brain, thereby giving relief. It's important not to use a TENS device without the supervision of your physician or physical therapist.

Acupuncture

Acupuncture is commonly applied for relieving pain caused by many illnesses and diseases. Acupuncture also helps the body to re-adjust its energy flow and as such, works to repair as well as alleviating pain.

Researchers have found that acupuncture can help increase bone density as much as 8.8%. Plus, their research showed that acupuncture can help increase the levels of osteocalcin, which is a biomarker of bone formation, by up to 30.9%.

Biofeedback

This technique helps people cope with pain, as it teaches them how to use their own body's responses to alleviate the stress and pain caused by osteoporosis.

During biofeedback sessions, sensors are attached to the body to measure the temperature of the extremities, heart rate and muscle tension.

Biofeedback sessions are performed under the supervision of a health care provider, cardiologist or urologist. Biofeedback can also be used in conjunction with cognitive-behavioral therapy.

Emotional Freedom Technique

EFT practitioners believe that when unhealthy habits, past traumas, unhappy memories and any other negative emotions are stored in the body, a disruption in its energy flow begins to occur.

This circumstance increases the incidence of many diseases that bring about pain and discomfort, including osteoporosis. Using EFT, or Emotional Freedom Techniques, the person will be able to help correct these energy imbalances, and healing can start to take place.

Realizing that osteoporosis is the cause of much of their pain comes as a shock to many newly diagnosed patients. Several methods exist to manage osteoporosis pain, so choose one or more that best suits your own particular set of conditions.

Diet for Osteoporosis

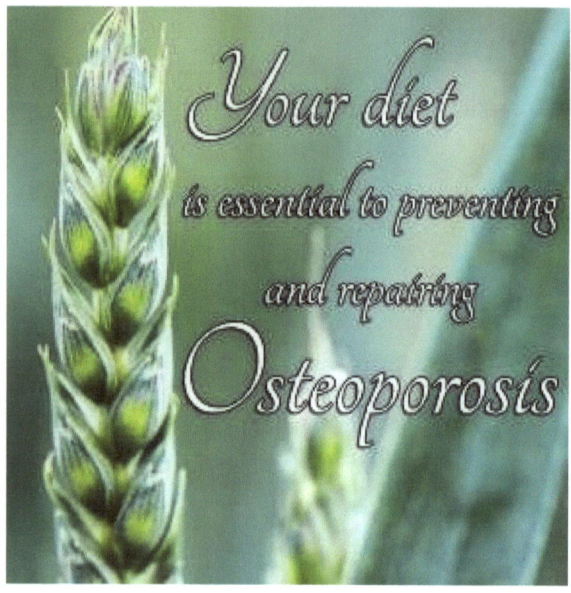

Osteoporosis has been nicknamed "the silent thief". Bone loss occurs incrementally without our being aware of it. Osteoporosis often presents without symptoms and can happen to anyone, although older women are statistically over-represented.

Osteoporosis seems like a new "disease", but there is little doubt it has always existed in humankind. Due to improved diagnostic capabilities and understanding of the processes involved in bone degeneration and regeneration, there is a seeming explosion in the rates of detection of the condition.

While our "sit-down" lifestyle may be a contributing factor, there is no doubt that diet is a huge factor in bone and skeletal health. There are also other preventative measures, such as getting adequate exercise and sunlight.

Diet is, however, almost always the single aspect of our lives that we can most influence and take responsibility for. There is increasing recognition that if we do not pay attention to our diet during our younger years, we may be more susceptible to the effects of osteoporosis in our later years.

Undoubtedly, following a diet for osteoporosis prevention is a smart move. This does not mean looking for a great or wonderful 'osteoporosis diet', however there are a variety of foods we can incorporate into our diets that can help prevent osteoporosis from happening, or at the very least, reducing its impact.

On the flip side, there are foods to avoid since these may interfere with absorption levels of important vitamins and minerals, or even cause them to be expelled from the body.

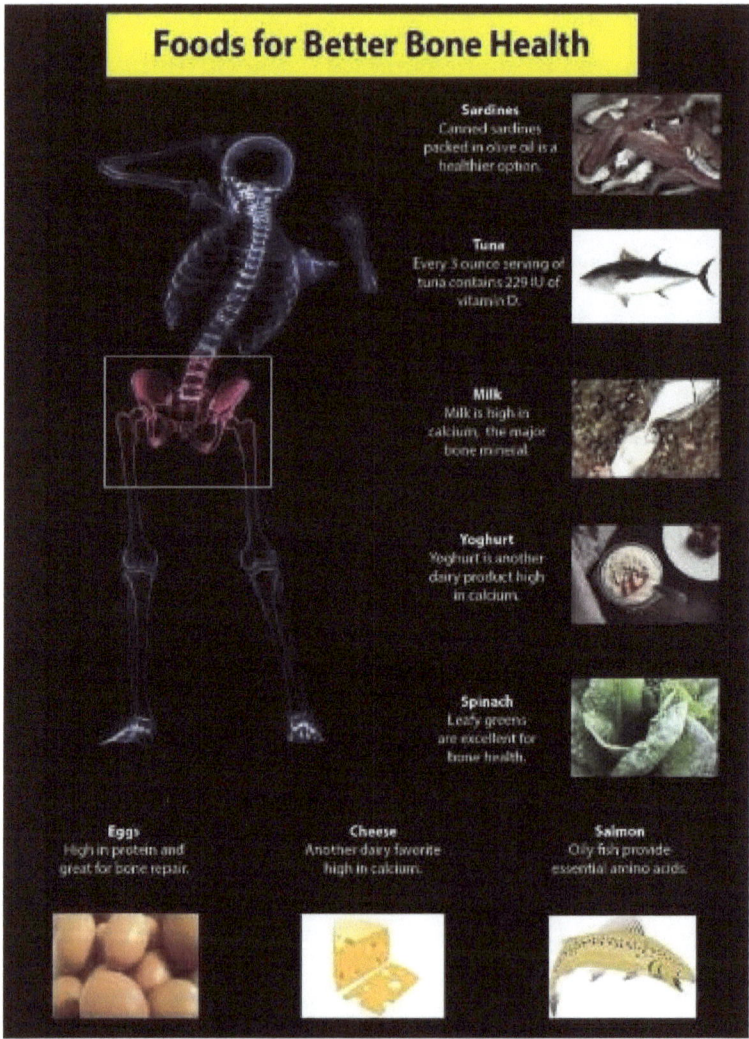

Foods to Eat

Calcium and magnesium are the two big 'macro' nutrients required to build healthy bone and maintain bone density.

Calcium Rich Foods

Conventional recommended dietary sources of calcium have had a great focus on dairy products, because they contain large amounts of calcium. However, recent research makes strong claims that the calcium obtained from vegetable sources such as leafy green vegetables is more effectively absorbed and utilized than that from dairy sources.

Calcium rich foods such as yogurt, milk and cheese are great dairy choices. Excellent non-dairy food sources include: lettuce, green tea, green peas, parsley and oats and lemons.

Lemons additionally contain trace minerals which are also essential for maintaining bone health. They are also high in Vitamin C, which increases overall calcium absorption.

Sweet potatoes, Atlantic sardines, pumpkins and pink salmon are other positive choices.

Magnesium Rich Foods

In order for your body to utilize the calcium you also need magnesium. In the past, dietary recommendations for osteoporosis prevention focused almost solely on calcium. Current research recognizes that intake of calcium is quite often adequate, but that calcium is not being properly utilized due to a lack of necessary complementary minerals and vitamins.

The biggest limiting nutrient is often magnesium, as it far more common to be deficient in magnesium than calcium. Magnesium rich foods include leafy green vegetables, brazil nuts, almonds and other delicious nuts and seeds, avocados, bananas and beans and lentils.

There are of course other foods rich in calcium and/or magnesium, so you are not limited to those mentioned above.

What Should You Avoid

Anyone with an interest in preventing or overcoming osteoporosis needs to be aware that consuming salt, soft drinks, caffeine and alcohol in excess is detrimental to bone health.

A high sodium diet can trigger the kidneys to excrete calcium before it can be utilized by the body. Caffeine too can cause the body to expel calcium. Tea contains caffeine in much smaller amounts, so switch to drinking tea if possible.

Prevention Is Always Better Than Cure

Following a healthy diet for osteoporosis prevention is probably the most effective action you can personally take to prevent this condition from impacting your future life. Certainly, there are other factors, but a healthy lifestyle is the best medicine in preventing bone loss. It is also the area over which you have the most control.

Osteoporosis and Bone Building

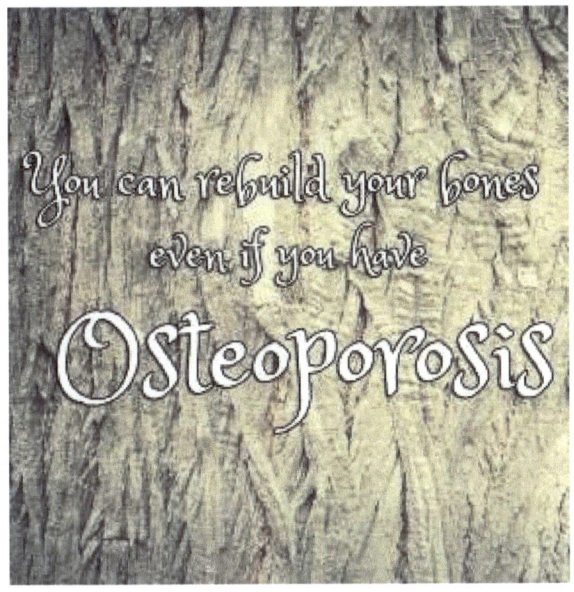

Weight bearing exercises are excellent for building strong, healthy bones! This is not news. Regular exercise promotes better health and reduces risks of being diagnosed with many diseases, including osteoporosis.

For most people, the words 'regular exercise' often brings to mind activities such as brisk walking or jogging. These activities are indeed beneficial for improving overall health, maintaining skeletal integrity, elevating the heart rate and for releasing toxins through perspiration.

However, few people realize that as we age strength training may prove to be more beneficial than aerobic exercises, especially for bone building.

Strength Training Works to Preserve Muscle Strength and Bone Density

For people aged 50 and above, strength training plays a crucial role in maintaining healthy bones.

Many studies show that engaging in aerobic exercises alone is not enough to preserve a person's muscle strength, bone density, posture and balance. Those who do not engage in strength training are at a higher risk of becoming less functional due to a decline in bone density and muscle strength.

Strong muscles help support the skeleton, even when osteoporosis is present. When both systems are weak the risk of bone damage through fractures is greatly increased.

Strength training can therefore greatly reduce the risk of fractures cause by osteoporosis. This is because strength training works two body systems at the same time. The strength training itself builds muscle. This helps maintain correct posture, increases dexterity and mobility, and protects the skeleton.

Strength Training for Better Bone Health

The weight-bearing aspect of the exercise prompts your body to rebuild bone loss. Weight training places 'natural stress' on your bones which encourages the additional development of bone-forming cells. This has a positive bone-building effect on the whole skeleton, as opposed to muscle-building, which tends to improved only the muscle group being stressed.

Unless a weight-bearing requirement is placed on the skeleton, there is no impetus to lay down bone growth. As there is an ongoing cycle of bone degeneration, unless it is replaced, osteoporosis is the result.

On the other hand, inactivity is one of the many factors that contributes to the reduction of bone mass, by as much as 1% each year once an individual reaches the age of 40. That may not sound much, but it quickly adds up in later years!

Strength Training and Body Weight Approaches

Strength training may include using free weights such as barbells or dumbbells, or elastic bands that allow you to improve the flexibility of your legs and arms.

It also includes ankle weights and vests along with other types of special exercises that make use of your body weight to simulate as well as develop resistance against gravity. The use of weight machines, resistance bands and free weights can help preserve and increase one's muscle strength and mass.

Starting Your Strength Training

Some people are hesitant about trying any types of strength training for fear of developing body aches and pains. The most important thing to keep in mind is to start very slowly, maintain consistency and pay attention to keeping proper form during strength training exercises.

Use very light weights to begin. Low weights will not put undue strain and stress on bones and joints. Don't risk causing fractures by going too heavy too soon.

If you have some degree of osteoporosis and your muscles are undeveloped due to inactivity, your bones are at risk if you over-estimate your ability.

Move slowly, steadily and methodically. Do not jerk, lunge or twist while using weights. Move the limb through only one plane of movement at a time, do not perform compound actions that cause twisting as this will place excess pressure on joints.

Work within your current limits and gradually progress into increasing levels of difficulty to avoid injuries. Starting any form of strength training with small weights and for only ten to fifteen minutes a day, should not cause any problems.

Beginners may expect to see the results of a healthier body after one or two months, and although you won't see your bones building back up, you will be making positive steps to rebuild bone instead of losing more. Improvements to muscle strength and tone will provide visible positive feedback to encourage you to continue.

With persistence, you will find yourself having better flexibility, less muscle aches, less joint pains and feeling freer in your movements.

It is possible to experience some muscle soreness during the first few weeks of training. Learn the difference between pain and discomfort and rest for a day or two if needed.

If you do notice abnormal pains, talk to your doctor or visit a clinic immediately. Be mindful of any swelling that could indicate a fracture, even of a small bone such as in the foot or hand.

Side Effects of Osteoporosis Medications

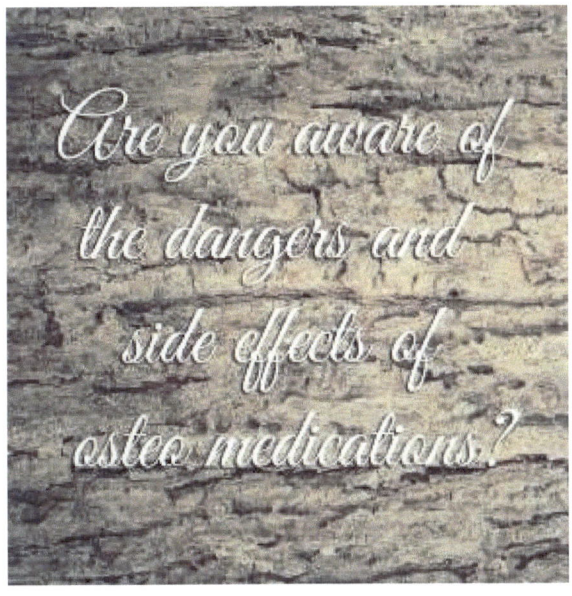

Individuals with osteoporosis suffer from a weakening of their bones which can make them more susceptible to fractures. This weakening occurs when bone replacement does not keep pace with bone degeneration.

Ideally, this process would result in perfect replacement, however, as we age, for various reasons, this is often not the case. Genetic factors and lifestyle causes such as indulgent diets and lack of exercise contribute to bone density loss, which is termed osteoporosis.

When osteoporosis is diagnosed, medical practitioners will offer advice regarding steps individuals can take to help arrest the progress of the condition.

However, doctors are acutely aware that many people will not take their advice regarding changes to lifestyle such as increased exercise and dietary changes.

Therefore, it is standard practice for many doctors to attempt to deal with the issue by prescribing certain medications. Broadly speaking, the function of these medications is not to encourage bone growth, but rather to inhibit the natural cycle of bone degeneration.

Unfortunately, these medications do come with side effects and associated health risks.

Severe Bone Pain

Some warnings have been issued by a group of researchers, cautioning individuals who have been prescribed with certain osteoporosis drugs, especially the bisphosphonates, to be aware of the potential to cause necrosis of the bone. This is an extremely painful and disfiguring condition.

The U.S. Food and Drug Administration has issued the same warning to additional drugs such as alendronate and risedronate due to these medications being reported to have caused intense bone pain in certain individuals.

Unusual Thighbone Fracture

Certain osteoporosis drugs which have been prescribed to prevent bone breakage, have actually been linked to rare cases of thighbone fractures, according to a report in the New York Times.

Some reports stated that women's bones were found to be snapping like twigs and splintering. Another concern was that cases of bone breakage were occurring without any serious falls or trauma to cause these types of fractures.

These studied groups of women were in their 50's and their bones were diagnosed at a stage of pre-osteoporosis, meaning their bones had not reached a super fragile phase at that point.

Further studies additionally revealed that these thighbone fractures from patients taking these drugs were quite unusual since they happened in the long bone portion of the thigh. Normal thighbone fractures typically occur close to a person's hip socket. An added complication of mid-thigh fractures is a longer healing time, due to a reduced blood supply in this area.

Osteonecrosis of the Jaw

Bisphosphonate treatments have become a growing concern as these drugs are often prescribed to individuals who have osteoporosis. Use of bisphosphonate treatments has been linked to osteonecrosis of the jaw.

This complication poses a serious threat as it can lead to the destruction of a person's jaw. It is becoming common practice for dentists to ask patients if they are taking bisphosphonate medication, and if so refusing to undertake some dental procedures.

Atrial Fibrillation

Research has shown that individuals taking Fosamax to strengthen bones can increase the potential for atrial fibrillation or chronic irregular heartbeat. Alendronate is the generic version of this drug. Studies reveal that women who have been taking Fosamax were found to have their risk of experiencing atrial fibrillation increased by up to 86% compared to those who have never had any alendronate or Fosamax medications.

Some of the issues linked to atrial fibrillation include: palpitations, fatigue, fainting and congestive heart failure.

There are more items on the list of potential side effects to be aware of, including esophageal and gastric inflammation, renal failure and reduced blood calcium. Eye inflammations are also among the reported side effects of osteoporosis medications.

Those who still feel that the benefit outweighs the risk as far as achieving better bone health via the use of these drugs need to be informed so that they are prepared for the possible adverse effects that may occur.

It is important to be aware that osteoporosis can be greatly mitigated with effective diet and self-care. Before taking any medications for osteoporosis, please do your research thoroughly. There are many side effects from these drugs and none are pleasant.

Final Thoughts

In this book, we have read how about what osteoporosis is, what causes it, its symptoms, some ways to reverse bone density loss and how to prevent it in the first place. We also talked about some supplements that might be beneficial depending on your circumstances, how diet affects or reduces bone density.

One very important factor we also discussed was the importance of "weight-bearing" exercise, as it spurs bone growth which can help replace what was lost. And finally, we read about possible side effects that some osteoporosis medications can cause.

As with many other types of conditions, lifestyle choices can make a huge difference. Smoking, drinking to excess, being sedentary are all bad choices and will speed up bone density loss. It makes no sense to do everything else right if you counteract it with an unhealthy lifestyle.

Unfortunately, unlike other conditions, once you have low bone density, you can't just take a pill and make it all better. Yes, we talked about some things that can be done to reverse the effects of bone density lost, but the best road to take is doing what you can to prevent the loss in the first place.

My hope is that you will continue to digest all the information in this book, re-read parts if you must and adjust your life the best you can to keep the density you still have and try to build back some of what you have lost.

Otherwise, you could fall victim to a fall resulting in a hip fracture. Many do not recover to the point of where they are independent and can take care of themselves anymore and are confined to an assisted living facility. Doing all the things in this book could prevent that from happening or at least stall it off for as long as possible.

Ron Kness

Other Relevant Books by This Author

If you would like to read more relevant books about this topic, here is a list of the CreateSpace links, titles and descriptions from this author:

https://www.createspace.com/6396809

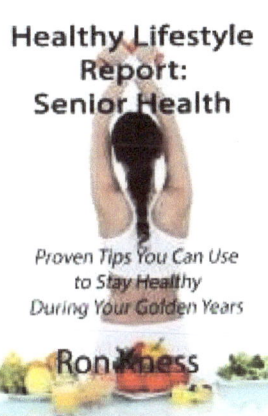

Healthy Lifestyle Reports: Senior Health: Proven Tips You Can Use to Stay Healthy During Your Golden Years

We live in a world where we want everything immediately. From having fast food restaurants on every corner, the ability to shop from our smartphones, to live streaming sports events, nearly everything we do is at our fingertips.

Besides not getting enough exercise from daily activities anymore, throw into the mix the plethora of junk food we consume (because it is quick) and it's no wonder that we as a nation continue to get more and more overweight and obese.

So instead of walking to the store, or walking around the mall for a few hours, we order our groceries online and buy new clothes and furniture with a few clicks on our computer or smartphones.

Now, instead of burning calories prepping for and cooking a healthy family dinner, we call up the pizza guy or swing by a McDonald's and pick up a cheap and unhealthy meal for the family. Convenience may seem nice but it comes with a price – obesity, heart-related diseases, Type II diabetes and an early death.

The health risks of being overweight and obese are frightening. The heavier you are, the higher your chance of getting Type 2 diabetes, having heart disease and high blood pressure, and getting certain cancers such as colon, kidney and breast.

However these health risks are reversible if you start now. Do you watch the T.V. show Biggest Loser? If so, then you know that most of the contestants come onto the ranch overweight and taking multiple medications for the conditions they have. After a few months on the ranch and several pounds lighter, most of them leave the ranch off of most, if not all, of their medications.

Everything they were trying to control with medication was directly related to them being overweight or obese. Once the weight was gone, the conditions disappeared.

According to the World Health Organization (WHO), 2.8 million people die each year due to the effects of being overweight or obese. Although the pharmaceutical companies' answer to the problem is to create more medicines, it's no secret that diet and exercise are vital in helping control this growing epidemic.

But today, it seems people would rather take a pill (due to the large advertising budgets of big pharma exulting how their newest pill will solve your health problem) then put in the work it takes to improve their health.

However, the shocking realization is that it is important we take responsibility for our own health and well-being.

By being informed (which this report will do) and taking an active role in your health, you can help decrease your chance of becoming another statistic.

https://www.createspace.com/6107842

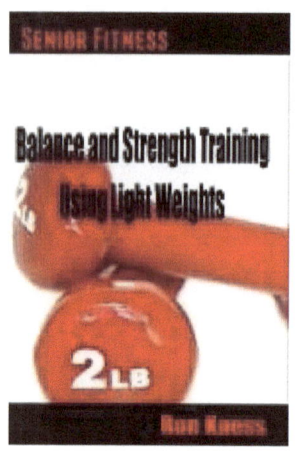

Senior Fitness - Balance and Strength Training Using Light Weights

As you age you notice that you are not as strong as before. Most of us simply chalk that up to the "natural" aging process. However, to fight the physical dangers of aging, strength is very important.

We are not talking about bodybuilding and packing on bulky muscles. What we mean is simply making your body stronger so that you don't become part of one of the following statistics ...

• Falls in those 75 or older contribute to 70% of accidental deaths.

• Respiratory issues such as COPD are the #3 cause of death for men and women 65 and older.

• 1 in every 3 people over 65 will fall each year. (Doctors are certain this number is drastically higher, since many falls are not reported because of embarrassment or concern over medical bills.)

• 1 in 5 Americans over 65 suffer from a lack of independence and reduced quality of life due to osteoporosis and/or diabetes.

• If you are 80 years or older, there is a 50% chance you will fall.

• As a senior citizen, if you fall once, you are 200% to 300% more likely to fall again.

• Heart disease impacts 26% of women and 37% of men 65 or older.

• Roughly 9,500 deaths in older US citizens each year are associated with falling.

• Even if you survive a fall as a senior citizen, you suffer a much greater functional decline in your ability to perform normal daily activities.

• Over 250,000 older Americans experience a fractured hip each year (research as of 1996, probably a larger number now due to aging of the US population)

• Over half of adults over 65 years of age are affected by arthritis.

• 1 in 4 seniors who fracture a hip die within 6 months as a result of that injury.

The real problem here is not the scary statistics just covered. The problem is that each and every one of the debilitating and even deadly issues we just mentioned can be positively impacted by simply lifting light weights, yet seniors are not strength training.

The following are the incredible benefits of simply lifting light weights a few times each week for seniors ...

• A feeling of self-esteem and self-confidence

• Improved circulatory system

• Lowered risk of heart disease

• Regulation of a naturally healthy body weight

• Light weightlifting is an effective way to treat and eradicate back pain

• You have fewer feelings of depression, anxiety and stress

• You strengthen your bones, naturally improving your ability to fight health issues like osteoporosis

• Light weightlifting is excellent for preventing and treating diabetes

• Arthritis sufferers experience fewer painful symptoms when they weight train regularly

• Your balance and flexibility are boosted, and joint pain is reduced.

By now you are probably sold on the fact that you need to be lifting light weights and strength training if you are over 50 years of age or older.

So, what's your next step?

https://www.createspace.com/6096479

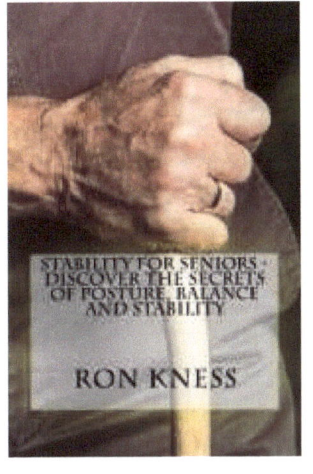

Stability for Seniors - Discover the Secrets of Posture, Balance and Stability

You may have noticed that some people in your neighborhood, who are in their 60s, have trouble walking and getting around. Yet, if you look at Sylvester Stallone, he is still muscular and in excellent shape. He is still directing and getting physical in his action movies. Stallone is in his sixties.

What about Arnold Schwarzenegger? His arms and muscles are bigger than those of men half his age. He doesn't seem to lack coordination or balance.

The dancer, Michael Flatley, is 57 and still dancing. The former model, Christie Brinkley, is sixty and she is as elegant and fit as ever.

What is the underlying reason here? Why these people are healthy and well-coordinated while you or others you may know are sickly, unfit or unable to move without assistance?

The answer is – the life choices we made.

Many people sacrifice their health in pursuit of their career. They are so busy making a living that they neglect to make a life.

The excuse that they do not have time to exercise is tossed about so frequently that they end up letting their health and fitness slide.

If you are not regularly active, you will have muscular atrophy over time. Your flexibility will decrease. Your core strength will diminish. As time progresses, you will be less limber and more rigid.

This is exactly how people age poorly. It's a process that has snowballed over time.

Only with regular exercise and a healthy diet can you have a body that is fit and has the ability to almost reverse aging.

If you have neglected your health for years and life seems to be a chore now because you can't get around without assistance, do not feel dejected.

You can remedy the situation. You can restore the strength, balance and stamina that you have lost. It is never too late to become what you might have been.

Your body will help you, if you help it.

This guide will show you exactly what you need to do to restore your balance, strengthen your core and give you the ability to live life to its fullest. Read how ...

About the Author

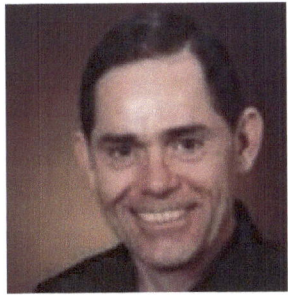

I grew up in Central Minnesota, where my parents owned and operated a fishing resort. Once out of high school I tried a couple of semesters of college, only to quit halfway through the Spring term; I decided at that time that college wasn't for me.

Then I decided to follow my father's previous occupation as an auto mechanic. I graduated from a two-year of vocational training course and worked as a mechanic for five years. While in vocational training, I decided to join the National Guard where I eventually ended up working full-time for 32 years.

So how does all of this relate to writing? In one of my leadership schools, the instructor, who was an English teacher at a juvenile detention center, presented writing to me in a whole new way - a way that started to develop my interest in working with words.

I eventually went back to college on the GI Bill while I was working and earned my Bachelor's degree in Business Administration. Taking a class or two per semester at night and on weekends took me seven years to complete my degree.

Fast forward about 40 years and I now have published over 75 books on Amazon for Kindle, CreateSpace and other publishing platforms.

Besides my own writing, I also ghostwrite ebooks, reports, articles, blogs and do Kindle conversions for clients on a variety of topics.

Today my wife and I are retired from our careers and live in Gold Canyon, AZ. I now write as a retirement business where you'll find me happily sitting in my office typing away on my laptop as I work on my next book or ghostwriting project . . . that is if we are not traveling on a cruise ship - our new-found mode of travel.

www.ingramcontent.com/pod-product-compliance
Lightning Source LLC
Chambersburg PA
CBHW050820290526
45792CB00001B/199